Be Successful By...

Follow Your Dreams

(It is Never Too Late to take Control over Your own Destiny)

By Neil Caine

Contents

Introduction

"Let us today seek to find that place within each of us where dreams are made, where our highest aspirations take shape. Let us confirm the power of our humanity by giving architecture and substance to the dreams we have for our nation so that the promised land of social and economic justice that is within our dreams will soon be within our sight."

-Dennis Kucinich

Each one of us has dreams and aspirations. Human beings have been exposed to the idea of dreams since the dawn of time. When you lay on the bed and close your eyes, you are constantly reminded of the aspirations and goals you want to achieve. Yet, the stresses of the world churning away make it difficult for most of us to accomplish those goals. However, all is not lost. There are ways one can successfully fulfill all their dreams and aspirations. Before diving into the said ways, we must explore why we have dreams and aspirations and how they differ from our peers. We have to determine why is it that fulfilling our dreams and aspirations makes us feel complete, filling a void within us?

Our dreams are the center of who we are. It is the essence of us as a person and the entire purpose of our being. Accomplishing our dreams gives us a sense of fulfillment. Ever since we were children, we had been told to stop daydreaming and be more practical. Our society has a tendency to separate our dreams and aspirations from practical life. Most people fall into this trap and leave their dreams and aspirations behind. They are conditioned to believe that nothing will come out of dreaming big. They couldn't be more wrong. Dreaming is the first step to achieving your aspirations and goals. When you dream, there is something to look forward to. You become happier; you shine as a person and are in a positive mood. Why? Because you have a purpose in life, and you know exactly what that purpose is. Just like how people brainstorm their ideas when marketing their products, we dream about our goals. Those who don't have dreams or aspirations are like plants that wither away without any sun or water. There is no spark in them. They float through their life without feeling deeply. Human beings are the only mammals that have aspirations. There is a reason why we were gifted with the ability to dream. To shun those dreams is doing a huge disservice to your humanity. Wanting something in life or dreaming about it is not a fleeting thought. You should pursue it. Dreams are what drives a person to be better and push themselves.

So then why is it so difficult to dream and/or follow them? It is because we have been programmed to think they are for children. We have been told that as you grow up, you should start living your life as opposed to dreaming. It is true we should live our life, but why can't we do both? Why can't we dream about the life we want, make it happen and then live it? Another problem our society has with dreaming is that it pulls us out of our comfort zone. Following your dreams requires effort, change and growth. It can be a bit uncomfortable initially, but like all good things, it takes patience and perseverance. When we try something new or enter unknown territory, the first thing we feel is fear. However, as you conquer that fear, you are exposed to a world of possibilities you didn't know about. Living your life with fear and worry will never make you go far. Living in your comfort zone will never help you grow as a person. Do you want to get out there and pursue your dreams? Or do you want to lock yourself in the house and be frustrated, irritated and angry? In the end, it is up to you which path you choose because only you will walk it and no one else. You will notice following your dreams will appeal to you more than the fears attached to them. The dreams and aspirations you have are your callings. Dreaming is equivalent to sowing the seeds. When you put effort into making those dreams into reality, you are essentially watering those seeds and helping them grow. Once your dreams turn into reality, you reap the fruits of your hard work, and it adds to your happiness. You feel lighter and positive. You begin enjoying everything in life. Your relationships improve, your productivity increases, you feel balanced, stress-free and whole as a person.

Dreams help us feel connected to our values. They lead us to a richer future and help us remember which direction to take our life in. They work as an engine fuel to help us drive our aspirations. When we muster up the courage to pursue our dreams, nothing can stop it. We are fully prepared to face all the challenges and live our lives with zero regrets. For those who think pursuing your dreams is a silly idea and that it is new-age hipster nonsense, then you are fooling yourself because all the greatest people who wanted the world to change for the better had a dream to do it.

Martin Luther King Jr. had a dream to eliminate racism from America. He had a dream to change the course of American history and make it more equal for everyone. He succeeded because he never stopped dreaming. He didn't allow anyone to stop him in his tracks. Had he backed down when people told him he was silly to think about changing history, America would be in a different place today.

Most accomplishments had been in the dream state for a long time before efforts were made to materialize it.

Why It's Never Too Late to Chase Your Dreams

We all have aspirations and dreams. We have thoughts on how we are going to achieve them, and we reflect on them. We imagine them and want them to turn into reality. But more often than not, we end daydreaming and let our dreams remain just dreams and nothing more. Most people have self-deprecating thought like:

- People are going to think I am insane
- If my dreams don't work out, I'll make a fool out of myself
- If my dreams won't work out, my life will be ruined
- I don't have enough time
- I am way too old to be pursuing my dreams
- I don't think I'd be able to pursue my dreams because I am not hardworking enough
- I am not smart
- I don't think I am ready
- I don't think I will ever be ready

The list of self-deprecating thoughts is endless. Even when we have positive thoughts about fulfilling our dreams, they always end with one word, "someday." That day is often forgotten, or people are so busy in their fast-paced life they forget about their dreams altogether. The point is it is never too late to fulfill your dream, whatever it may be. Don't allow your dreams to take a backseat, or when you are on your deathbed, regrets will get the better of you. Here are a few crucial reasons why you should never let go of the idea of chasing your dreams. For all you know, your dreams could have the potential of helping you reach self-actualization.

Nothing is Set in Stone

You must remember nothing is black and white. Just because you are comfortable and settled in your life with your current job doesn't mean you can't move things around in order to follow your dreams. The internalized idea about what we are supposed to do and who we are supposed to be in our society hinders our personal growth. It makes us part of a rat race even if we never wanted to compete. Some insecurities from your childhood could come up to the surface when you attempt to make your dreams into a reality.

Many people project their own fears and limit themselves from moving ahead in life. Don't allow the negativity and destructive beliefs hold you back from reaching your true potential. Dream big and celebrate your life.

Small Steps

Don't assume that to make a dream come true, you must take a huge step. Baby steps are an ideal way of reaching for dreams. If you keep thinking about doing big things, it will intimidate you, and you will pull back. For instance, note down your path of success in ten steps. Make sub-steps for each step. Also, make sure your initial steps are achievable so you don't get disheartened. Even if you accomplish only one step in a span of a couple of months, it will give you enough motivation to keep moving forward.

Reading books and articles about the law of attraction will help you. The law of attraction is when you attract what you want in life by thinking about it. If you constantly think about something negative, you will manifest negative events in your life and vice versa. Many people have undertaken manifestation techniques and found out that it works. This suggests that no matter where you are in life or how old you are, all it takes is your mindset. Our mind is a powerful organ. Once we set our mind to something, we achieve it without a doubt.

Regret Can be Avoided

Some time back, a book was published, a compilation of accounts of people's regrets when they were interviewed on their deathbeds. One of the most common regrets was not following the dreams. As we grow older, we may get accustomed to the life we are living. When everything is said and done, we will think about the things that could have made us happy, but we were too ignorant or too busy to do them. It can be a painful experience to realize you have run out of time. Everything comes and goes — lovers, friends, money, but time never waits for anyone. Take the opportunity you have been given in this world to chase what you want.

Securing Your Legacy

How you live your life has a big influence on your children, grandchildren and your family members. In a way, you're leaving behind a legacy. For instance, if you choose to follow your dreams, your children might do the same, and their children might follow suit. They might get the encouragement and motivation required to make it happen. If they see you rebelling against the norms of our society of fitting into a box, they will be comfortable forging their own path. You will be leaving behind a legacy that will aim high and live their life passionately. Thinking about leaving a lasting impression on the generations after your demise might help you chase your dreams more vigorously.

Chasing Your Dreams is a Step Forward Never Backwards

When you vow to chase your dreams, remember it means you are moving ahead in life. It never means you are losing out or putting your life on hold by pursuing something. This is often the excuse most people make. They say," Oh, I can't quit my job or put my life on hold on a whim. I know I have dreams, but I need to sort out other more pressing matters in my life." The thing is, if you live your life with that mindset, you will never get the time to pursue your dreams. There will always be one thing or the other that requires your attention. You don't have to quit your job or put your life on hold, but you can take out a few minutes of your day to think about how you will turn your dream into a reality. Sometimes what looks like taking a step backward actually helps you move forward and grow.

You will Get the Support

If you think you will be alone, you won't. No matter what you decide to do in the future, you will always have the support of your family and friends. If not, there will be someone who will believe in you. All you need to do is take a leap of faith. There will always be someone who will be there for you and support you through your journey. They will encourage you to be the best version of yourself. Don't forget that the world is full of possibilities. It is never too late to create something wonderful for yourself. It is never too late to chase after what your true calling is, and if you fail, pick up the pieces around you, dust off your pants and try again.

Things That Hold You Back From Chasing Your Dreams and Aspirations

Life struggles can get the better of you and hold you back when it comes to fulfilling your dreams. The pressure of our daily life and responsibilities wear us out so much we hardly get time or energy to think about our dreams, let alone chase them. There are a few common reasons why people hold back from pursuing what they want. To solve a problem, one must find what is causing it. Similarly, to stop holding ourselves back, we must recognize the reason we feel this way. And unfortunately, there is more than one reason that prevents us from moving forward.

Our Fears

Fear is the ultimate enemy of progress. It prevents a lot of people from pursuing their goals and makes them afraid to step out of their comfort zone. Fear is one of the most common reasons we hold ourselves back. Also, there are different types of fears, such as:

- Fear of being rejected
- Fear of experience humiliation and ridicule

- Fear of failing
- Fear of getting disappointed

Making Excuses

If you find yourself putting off things that could help you achieve your dream, it means you are making excuses. When you feel halted in life when it comes to your goal and aspirations, it is about time you determine what is causing it. If it is nothing external, it could be your attitude towards life. Maybe you are too afraid to pursue your dreams, and therefore, you are making excuses for it. People who want to achieve goals steer clear of excuses. Some of the common excuses people make are:

- I am too caught up with other things
- I don't think I am ready yet
- I am too old I don't have enough time
- I am too young, and I have plenty of time
- Avoid making excuses and try to get out of your comfort zone.

Procrastinating

This is similar to making excuses. Putting things off to next month or year or life is not good. This way, you will never be able to achieve your goals. It is true good things come to those who wait, but waiting to make efforts will never serve you. Once you do everything in your power to realize your dreams, then only you can wait. As mentioned earlier, time never waits for anyone, so procrastination will only hurt your chances of getting what you want.

Lack of Faith and Believe

A lack of faith in yourself and your ability to achieve greatness certainly holds you back. What we believe in our subconscious determines the action we will take in life. If we hold self-limiting thoughts, we will never be able to live our life to the fullest and do what we want.

Nothing can stop you. Only you have the power to hold yourself back from pursuing your goals.

No Focus

When you lose focus, it kills your chances of success. When we spread ourselves too thin, it makes us lose our focus. The effort we put into accomplishing what we want can be diffused by lack of focus. Take some time off your busy schedule and focus on your dreams. You don't have to put all your attention into them, but some level of focus is required if you want to be successful.

Instant Results

There are certain things that take a long time to accomplish. If you get impatient and expect instant results, you are in for a disappointment. It will do nothing but make you frustrated and discouraged. Everything in life takes time. Goals take a few months or even years to come to fruition, but the only people who can achieve their goals are people who never give up. You must remember that it won't happen overnight. Take your time to work on the goals, and don't give up. Even if you feel like it's not going anywhere, keep at it. If you want to get instant results to drive your motivation, take smaller steps. Maybe keep your initial goals to something that can be achieved in a matter of days instead of months or years. Once you list down smaller goals and accomplish them, it will be easy for you to be patient and work on bigger ones.

Lack of Vision

When we don't have a clear vision about an idea or goal, it never comes to fruition. It always helps to know what comes next in order to achieve your goals. It makes it a lot easier to take the necessary steps and reach the end. You could also share your ideas with others or write them down on a notepad. Every time you feel like you are steering away from your goals, read what you have written on the notepad to remind yourself. Friends and family can help you figure out the steps to help you reach your goals.

You should be able to visualize what you want in life and then take steps to make it happen. If you are unsure of your future goals, then try to figure that out. Finding your true purpose in life is the most fulfilling feeling ever.

Resources

One of the main things that hold us back from achieving our dreams is the lack of resources. Sometimes we have the determination but little to no resources. It is a legitimate barrier, but it all comes down to whether or not you are looking for a solution. Everybody has to deal with challenges in life; the main quality of successful people is their ability to find solutions to their problems. They never give up or sit with hands on their lap, waiting for a miracle to happen. Research your goals and work on accomplishing them by creating a feasible plan. Do what you can, and the rest will fall into place.

There Is No Consistency

It is important to be consistent when you want to get the results. For all tasks, keep in mind that consistency is key, and this is especially true when you want to keep progressing. Most successful people are consistent in their life, be it their nighttime routine, their work out routine or a set of habits that add positivity in their life. If you will like pursuing your goals one day and want to give up the next day, you will never be able to chase your dreams. Find your dream and work toward it consistently.

Mistakes People Make When Wanting to Fulfill Their Dreams

There are many mistakes people make when chasing their dreams. Some are mistakes they learn from, while others do nothing but hold them back. Identifying the mistakes that hold you back is the first step to solving them. Doing so will help you get back on track to making your dreams a reality. We tend to make excuses, being stuck in our daily routines, and take shortcuts, thinking we will reach our end goals regardless. However, most people fail to realize it is those very things acting as stumbling blocks in our journey. Here are a few crucial mistakes to avoid that get in the way of achieving your dreams.

Giving Up When Things Get Uncomfortable

When we start something new, a bit of nervousness is inevitable. Everybody has a fear of abandonment. If you are serious about fulfilling your dreams, you will have to put the fear behind you. When things get uncomfortable, you must persevere and move on ahead. When we go through uncomfortable or challenging situations, they help us grow as people. It aids our personal growth. Chasing your dreams might take an emotional toll on you, and that might stop you from taking the next step. You need to remember that good things require courage. You will eventually have to learn to deal with the problems. When someone learns how to drive a car, they have to be courageous, trust themselves, and push ahead. With experience, they will get the hang of it. Similarly, you have to push yourself harder.

Shortcuts

Another major mistake people make is depending on shortcuts to meet their goals. Taking shortcuts will never help you in the long-run. If you are looking for something that will make you be the first one in line without putting in any effort, you are in for a surprise. It doesn't work like that. You will have to find what you want to achieve, put in your blood, sweat, and tears, be true to yourself and your journey, and then only you will see success. To create a dream life, we must be willing to put in the work. If you want to launch a bakery store, you must know how to bake and practice baking different goods, such as cakes, breads, pastries, and so on. You can't open up a bakery store just because you baked a cake once at your niece's birthday party. A lot of time and effort is required for people to make it. Discipline is necessary for success. Also, remember there is always room for improvement. When chasing your dream, if you feel like you can go an extra mile, go for it. Stop taking shortcuts. There is no magic wand for making your dreams come true overnight.

Perfectionist

You don't have to wait for things to turn out to be perfect or wait for the stars to align. Most people tend to blame their circumstances for not being able to chase their dreams. Doing so is a huge mistake. If you want to accomplish your goals, you must take matters into your own hands and acknowledge that sometimes things won't work out. Yet, you have to keep moving forward.

You don't have to worry about doing everything perfectly. We live, and we learn. It means that even if you make a few mistakes, it will be a learning curve. It is all part of the process. For instance, if you want to start your own lifestyle blog, there will be a few hiccups in the beginning, but you will eventually get the formula and do well. Think about it; successful people didn't experience success overnight. They probably made a lot of mistakes, some that couldn't be easily fixed. As per Dr. Kerr L White, "Who said good judgment comes from experience and experience comes from bad judgment?"

Not Listening To Your Heart

The mind tends to overanalyze and worry about things, and the heart just wants us to take a dive with our eyes closed. Now, following your mind is not a bad thing. It is an important tool that helps us make informed decisions. However, sometimes we have to listen to our heart. When doing something we are not supposed, the heart will be the first one to give us a sign. Some people may not be able to tell, but the feeling of discomfort is there. Our mind tries to rationalize that moment after our heart guides us.

Waiting For Help

Will you be rejected for asking for help? Yes, more than you think. However, don't let this fear get in the way of asking for help. Sometimes, to achieve our dreams, we have to ask for help. We can't do everything in this world alone. The biggest mistake someone can make is not to ask their friends and family for support. This pride is the reason why so many people who set out to fulfill their dreams fail. You don't wait for people to extend a helping hand. Nobody knows what you go through. Therefore, reach out to people. You'd be able to differentiate between people who are your close friends and those who aren't. If one door closes, go in through the other. Others can give you a different perspective that could help you in your journey.

Don't Take it Personally

Some people judge, and that's a fact, but that doesn't mean you stop pursuing your dreams. Some people have nothing better to do than to care about what others are doing in their lives. Just because they couldn't amount to anything, they try everything in their power to bring others down. It has nothing to do with others but more to do with their own insecurities and fears. Do not allow others to rain on your parade. Turn a deaf ear to those who judge, feel happy and be proud of your achievements and journey.

Don't Give in to Negative Thought Patterns

Sometimes when things don't go our way, or there are delays in our goals, we can give in to a negative mindset. We could go down a negative spiral and victimize ourselves. This only hinders our progress. Instead of finding solutions to the obstacles in our journey, we tend to complain about them.

Suppose something doesn't work out; it's okay to feel negative. It's okay to cry and feel down, but then you have to pick yourself up again and move forward with full force. You shouldn't let a small stumbling block get in the way of your dreams. Be resilient.

Stop Comparing Yourself

Comparing ourselves to others' success is the worst thing you can do. Comparison leads to envy and jealousy. Instead of focusing on your own progress, you end up focusing on what the other person is doing. Doing so will prove detrimental to your own journey. Rather than obsessing over what the other person is doing, divert your focus on yourself and be grateful for who you are, how far you have come, what you have become, and how far you have the ability to go. Always keep a positive mindset and understand that everybody has their own path to walk on.

Trying to Seek Approval

Stop looking to others for validation. Your dream is your dream. It doesn't matter what others think. You have control of your life. If you wait for others' approval, you will never be able to reach your goals. You will keep on waiting and waste your precious time.

Mistakes to Avoid When Chasing Your Dreams

Chasing dreams is not easy, but there are some mistakes that can be avoided when you set out into the world. These mistakes can make it difficult for people to pursue what they want. Here are some mistakes to avoid when chasing your dreams.

Accept Your Reality

You have to recognize and accept your current situation. You may be in a good place right now and, therefore, may not want to budge but think of this as a starting point. Being in a good place is an excellent time to chase your dreams. No one can bring a change in your life except you. If you can't take major steps to pursue your dreams, then take small steps every day. For example, if you want to become a lawyer, but you have a good job as a manager at a company, start looking into part-time MBA courses in the universities in your city. Simply searching for a course online counts as a step forward. The mistake would be to wait for the opportunity to knock at your door instead of going out and grabbing it.

Let the Past Go

Dwelling in the past is never a good idea. If there was a time you tried pursuing your dreams and it didn't work out doesn't mean the same is going to happen again. You must move on from the past. Think of your past experiences as a learning curve. Sometimes going through hardships is exactly the jolt we need to pursue our life's true purpose. Think about it; you may have learned something in the past that could be useful to you either now or in the future. It could be a different mindset. Allow the painful memories and self-debilitating thought patterns to leave your system by thinking positively.

Don't Let Failure Get in the Way

Disappointments and failures are part of life, accept them, learn from them, and launch right ahead towards your destiny. Malcolm X stated, "Children have a lesson adults should learn, to not be ashamed of failing, but to get up and try again. Most of us adults are so afraid, so cautious, so 'safe,' and therefore so shrinking and rigid and afraid that it is why so many humans fail. Most middle-aged adults have resigned themselves to failure."

When you allow failure to crush you, you adopt a defeatist attitude. This attitude makes you miss all the important opportunities. The world moves on while you are sitting in the corner, feeling sorry for yourself and thinking about the disappointments and failures in your life.

Avoid Stalling

Stalling your dreams is the worst mistake you can make. Waiting for the right time, the right resources, and the right tools, and so on is never a good idea. If you want something, you make it happen. Otherwise, you will just be delaying your journey. One thing that never comes back or waits for us is time. Therefore, think about how you utilize it. This quote by Chris Burkmen perfectly describes why we should avoid stalling "Beginning is scary, exciting, terrifying, and all things amazing. Begin even when you're not sure...What do you have to lose?"

Do whatever you want but do it now so that you have no regrets later in life.

Don't Seek Approval

Don't wait for people around you to praise you for doing something or applaud your dreams. Keep your head down and go for it. Everyone's perspective is different. It may not resonate with you, and they may not be on the same page as you. When someone encourages you to take it but besides that, do what you have to do to achieve your dreams.

Don't Neglect Your Health

A lot of us underestimate the value of our health. We have been given only one body so we must take care of it. Without our health, nothing matters. If you are not fit and healthy, you won't be able to pursue your dreams. Therefore, eat healthy, work out, go out for walks for some fresh air, practice mindfulness, and do meditation. Treat your body with the love and respect it deserves, and then go on chasing your dreams. A healthy body means a healthy mind. If your mind is healthy, you will be in a headspace to work more efficiently towards your dreams. The strategy you create will be solid, and achieving your dreams will become easier.

Regrets of Those Who Gave Up on Their Dreams and Aspirations

What is regret? It is the pain, sadness, or disappointment of not being able to do something or a failed attempt. It is a feeling that stays with you long after the event has passed. Some people regret eating a chocolate cake on the weekend, some people regret not waking up for work early, and others regret gaining weight. However, there are those who take their regrets to their graves. It's those people who gave up on their dreams and aspirations. There have been countless accounts of people on their death beds expressing their regrets for not following their own path and fulfilling their dreams either because other people told them it was a stupid idea or they didn't want to get out of their comfort zone.

Of all the deepest regrets people have on their deathbeds, giving up their dreams was the first one. When people realize they only have a few days to live, they think about all those times and chances they had to make it happen. To live their life the way they wanted. This is why it's so important to do what your heart desires and never holds back because of others. These are the most common regrets related to not pursuing dreams.

I Wish I Didn't Work All the Time

This is perhaps one of the most common reasons why people don't pursue their dreams. They get comfortable in their lives. Some people regret being the only breadwinners in the family because it hinders their chances of being able to do something for themselves. Even when people get the chance, they are too afraid to take that leap of faith. Time doesn't wait for anyone, and once they realize what they missed, it is too late. People get jobs and earn money to pursue what they want.However, if they can't utilize that money to follow their dreams, all those years of breaking their backs go to waste.

It is crucial to slow down and evaluate our life from time to time. It gives us room to think about what we may or might have missed and taken actions accordingly. When we are too busy with our lives, we forget about the golden opportunities that we might have in front of us.

I Wish I Had the Courage

Courage is another reason why most people don't follow their dreams. It takes bravery and perseverance to drop everything and launch towards our aspirations. A lot of people work hard for years to build a safe cocoon where they can live comfortably and retire. It takes a courageous and brave person to break out of that cocoon and metamorphosis into a beautiful butterfly.

Most people aren't comfortable facing difficulties and challenges and would choose not to if given a choice, even at the cost of their dreams. They suppress their feelings, emotions, and aspirations and follow everybody else in the rat race. This can cause a lot of bitterness and resentment in some people. It can also ultimately affect relationships with their loved ones.

I Wish I Had Asked For Help

Pride and ego become the ruiner of some people. It is what stops them from reaching out to their friends and family for help and support. Human beings were never meant to do things alone in this world. The foundation of our species is togetherness, camaraderie, and teamwork. It's how we have made scientific revolutions, and it's how we came out of the caves and reached our potential. Asking others for help when you want to pursue your dreams is not something that is frowned upon. If anything, it is encouraged. Because helping your friends today means you will be there for your friend tomorrow. Being there for each other is what builds life-long friendships and relationships. When our health fades, it is our family and friends who take care of us and help us. Support from friends and family is a lot more important than wealth. Money might be crucial for fulfilling some dreams. However, ultimately, what matters is who you know and what they can do to help out.

Reach out to your friends for help and encourage them to do the same. Everybody needs help and support from time to time. It is what keeps this world going, and it is what helps our species flourish.

I Felt Misunderstood

A lot of people drop what they are doing because other people fail to understand their vision. The societal norms may hinder a person from pursuing their dreams and they may have given in to the people around them. More often than not, it is the discouragement we get from the people around us, which brings us down. In this situation, we must persevere. We have to keep moving forward regardless of what other people say.

I Wish I Hadn't Settled

The biggest regret is not being able to get out of the comfort zone. People regret settling for something they didn't want because they got too comfortable. People fail to realize that following dreams and pursuing something new is not easy. It can get uncomfortable, it can be difficult and there may be times when you want to quit. However, nothing good in life comes easily. That's why settling often leads to regret down the line because you had that chance but you were too afraid to take it. In this case you can't blame anyone else but yourself. That's the part that hurts the most.

I Wish I was More Flexible

Life happens and things change. If you wanted to become a stand-up comedian but could only get free gigs in small comedy houses or restaurants doesn't mean you will never make it. You have to be flexible and work your way around the hardships. Successful people don't succeed overnight. There is a lot of hard work and hours of sleepless nights involved. Most successful comedians performed free shows for months, maybe even years before getting discovered. Someone being too proud to adjust their goals or the things they had to do to achieve their dreams may regret it down the line. When you want something, nothing in this world should be able to stop you.

I Wish I Knew What I Wanted

Sometimes the dreams we want to pursue are perhaps not what we want deep inside. As a result, we get bored and stop pursuing it. Not only do we stop pursuing the dream we thought we wanted to achieve, we stop looking for our life's purpose. Sometimes achieving our dreams take longer than usual. Life may become monotonous and if you don't know exactly what you want, you get bored and drop the idea altogether. You go back to living your life the way you did before wanting to pursue your dreams.

I Wish I had Believed in Myself

When we have low self-esteem it can be easy for us to get swayed in another direction. It can be easy for other people to influence our decisions and lead us astray from our path. If you believe in your abilities no one can make you give up your dreams. Even the most secure people struggle with others not appreciating them. People give up on their dreams because they stop believing in themselves. They are afraid of failing and wasting everybody's time, including theirs.

Guarantees

Some people regret waiting for guarantees in order to pursue their dreams. Life is unpredictable. You can never have a 100% guarantee of how a certain situation will turn out. At the end of the day it's our faith in the universe and ourselves that keeps us going. There is no guarantee especially when you set out into the world to pursue your dreams. The thought of putting a job with a steady income at risk is scary. It can make a lot of people back off from pursuing their dreams.

Listening to Negativity

Some people regret paying attention to negativity oozing from the pores of people around them. Toxic people don't rain on your parade because they care about you or fear you are making a mistake by chasing a dream. They simply feel too insecure to witness another person launching towards greatness. A lot of people listening to the negative voices lose out on the opportunity to fulfill their dreams.

I Regret Giving Up After One Try

Failure is part of life. It is what helps you grow and learn important lessons. For instance, an actor might bomb in their audition, but they keep trying. Top actors experience more rejection than an average person but it never stops them from trying over and over again. Some people may have given up after one obstacle or failure in pursuing their dreams. That becomes their biggest regrets.

They Don't Want to Work Hard

There are some people who want all the rewards without working for them. They want things to magically happen for them and when they don't they simply sit back either wait for things to go their way or give up. That is not how life works. Everything in this world has to be earned. When you work hard you earn the reward. Everything takes time to come to fruition. When pursuing a dream, a lot of people focus on the end result instead of enjoying the process. Therefore, when they don't see the end results after only a few weeks or months, they give up. When everything is said and done, they look back and regret not standing their ground.

Change Destructive Habits

Change is a difficult process. It is time consuming and you have to spend a good chunk of your time engaging in self-awareness and self-evaluation. You have to really dig deeper into your psyche and thought process to identify destructive habits and then work on changing them. Here are a few ways to change habits that hinder you from progressing forward in life.

Feeling the Pain

Sometimes when we are comfortable in our life, we don't feel the need to change things in our life. Some people take inspiration from others around them, while others need to go through painful events in their lives to be able to make the necessary changes. If you are going through a painful phase in your life, allow yourself to feel it fully. Don't suppress your emotions because it will only make things worse for you. Try to understand what is causing the pain, what is the reason behind it? After that write all your emotions down. Now that you have identified the problem, it is time to solve it.

Eliminate Shame From Your Life

Feeling shame is one of the major self-destructive behaviors. Saying things such as "I am not a good person" instead of saying "what I did was bad" is indulging in shame. It leads to even more self-destructive behaviors. You would start believing you are a bad person and continue doing bad things. It can be a vicious cycle that can be hard to break. You can break the cycle by replacing harmful behaviors with healthy ones. Positive behaviors are the antithesis of shame and help foster pride. You could do that by, for instance, being completely honest. Instead of going down the route of telling a white lie, thinking it's harmful, tell the truth. Take responsibility for your mistakes, make lifestyle changes, and work on your mental health. All these things will help you move forward in life.

Be Prepared

Unhealthy and destructive habits can be difficult to see. Sometimes it can take you years to find out what triggers us. Therefore, constant self-evaluation is a great way of finding out what your destructive habits are and then take steps to work on them. Being prepared ahead of time is going to make things a lot easier for you when you decide to pursue your dreams. If your goal is to start working out, plan ahead by searching for affordable gyms in your area, look for healthy meal recipes to facilitate your work-out journey, and so on. Be mindful of your thought patterns and feelings. Planning ahead will equip you to be able to come up with better coping strategies when things don't go as planned.

Face the Problems

One of the main issues with changing destructive habits is sweeping the problem under the rug. When we let the problem fester by avoiding it for too long, it can be difficult for us to cope with it. That's why we should face our problems head-on. The more we distract ourselves from the problem, the more it gets worse. You should look at the problem, acknowledge it, and then understand how you can change it.

Take Small Steps

Once you have decided to eliminate destructive habits from your life, start small. It is tempting to start making major changes right away, but it will be difficult for you to commit to those changes. Take baby steps, and then work your way up. Be realistic. Pick one change and then stick to it. Don't try to add another step until you are sure you won't forget about the last one. For example, if you want to incorporate healthy eating in your routine, start with eating one fruit or one vegetable every day. Then slowly, replace your breakfast with something healthy, and then add 10 minutes of exercise, so on and so forth.

Stay Committed

The only way to commit to your goals is by starting small and being consistent. Committing to doing something is a huge responsibility. It is not easy. A lot of people start something but hardly get to the finish line. The best way to stay committed to something is by getting support from your loved ones. Ask your friends and family to hold you accountable for the things you promised yourself to do. Maybe join an accountability group, or announce your goal on social media. Keep a journal and write your goals down. Set a timeline for yourself and ask your loved ones to keep reminding you.

Not Believing In Yourself

When you set out to follow your dreams, there will be doubts and obstacles, but you must persevere in the face of adversity. Learn to believe in yourself. Have faith in yourself and your abilities.

Take Failure as a Learning Curve

Failure is a part of life. Failing at something doesn't mean you can't do something. It is an opportunity for you to learn from your mistakes. You should learn what works best and what doesn't. Failing means you had the courage to try something new. Don't use up your energy in negative self-talk. Improve yourself by changing things up. When it comes to destructive habits, you won't be able to get rid of them all at once. You will fail multiple times, and you will feel like giving up sometimes. It is a natural part of the change.

Try to find what triggers your destructive habits and then change your negative attitude towards not being able to fix them. For instance, if you want to quit smoking, don't beat yourself up for smoking every day. Even if you quit for a few days and start again, don't give up. Assess the situation, learn from your mishaps, pick up the pieces, and move forward.

Aspirations That Will Help You Design Your Life

You must have noticed when marketers pitch their ideas for products, they don't simply get out of bed and then write something on a piece of paper. They design a full-fledged plan, outlining everything they will use to promote the product. They write down the details step by step and then present it to the CEOs. Similarly, if you want to achieve something in your life, you must make a plan and then work towards it. You need to understand what steps you will be required to take to fulfill your dream. While you are making the plan, there would be some hiccups that you might need to deal with.

If you are confused about where to start, here are a few steps to help you take the first step.

Be Clear About What You Desire

First and foremost, figure out what you want. Ask questions, contemplate, and take your time to understand where you stand in your life. Finding out what you want is the core of designing the life you want for yourself. People in our society are overwhelmed with so many thoughts, inputs, opinions, and beliefs coming from other people. Before doing anything, they worry about what others will think about them, how society will view them. They worry about being judged for pursuing their dreams, and so they change their life's direction to suit others' narrative of what life should be. When we are judged for our choices, it becomes easy for us to lose touch with our life's purpose. When we lose touch with what we want, we end up living an unfulfilled life. It is important to seek clarity before devising a plan.

You can attain clarity by meditating or keeping a journal. Note down all your feelings and aspirations. This type of mapping will help you forge a clear path for the future.

Creating a Solid Plan

After you have figured out what you want, it is time to create or design a plan. The plan will involve small steps or goals at the initial stage. Completing smaller steps will be easier in the beginning and will encourage you to move forward.

You may want to jump to completing bigger tasks but think about it when architectures design a building, they start with something small. It is the small parts of the building that come together to form a huge complex. Remember, details are important. The detailed structure of a building is what makes it a building. One of the main reasons they are unable to fulfill their dreams is because they don't want to put in the time and effort. It may be tedious, but it's all worth the effort in the end.

Take out a bit of time from your busy schedule and create a plan to make your dreams come true. Imagine yourself as an artist creating an art piece that is your life. You must put all the energy, faith, and hard work into your plan.

Be Open-Minded

Designing your life the way you want is a life-long journey. That is something you can't achieve overnight. There may be several challenges and disappointments in your journey, but that doesn't mean you should give up. Continue moving forward. Be open-minded because you may need to take another route to reach your final destination.

You may put all your energy into a certain plan and find out that it didn't work. That's why you should be flexible. Some aspects of our lives are constantly changing and evolving.

What you planned a few months ago, may not work now. That's why doing plenty of research into your dream and how to go about it is best.

In the face of adversity, you may not fulfill your dreams should you choose to carry out the original plan. You could consider new future opportunities.

Sometimes, we think we want something, but the universe has other plans for us. Somewhere along the line, you may find another calling. What you decided to achieve 3 years ago may not be of interest to you anymore, or you might feel like it doesn't serve you anymore.

Learn to Say "No"

You should be able to draw clear boundaries between yourself and the people around you. If one weekend you have decided to spend time at home, figuring out your life, and you get an invitation to go out, say no, no matter how much your friends force you to get out. Spending time with yourself is an essential part of self-discovery, and self-discovery helps us truly understand what we want from life. It is okay to not do anything and be with your thoughts. We are taught that if we aren't busy, we are wasting away our life. If you are always busy, you will never be able to work on your dreams. Remember busy is not a default way of living.

Ignore Everyone and Achieve Your Dreams

To successfully achieve your dreams, you should ignore a few things. These things are not necessarily easy to evade and tend to get in the way. Having dreams is the easy part; what's difficult is achieving them. Not listening to people and doing what is required takes time, effort, and commitment. Dreams require sacrifice in other aspects of life. Dreaming requires you to envision something that hasn't happened yet but you want it to happen. In the process, there will be a lot of bumps and roadblocks. You will experience many problems related to money, time, resources, and location. Instead of giving up, you must keep moving forward. You have to navigate through the rough waters and safely reach the shore. Nothing in this world is impossible. What matters is how you go about it. The most important thing to do when it comes to achieving your dreams is ignoring what others have to say to you.

Ignore Your Colleagues

If you observe your friends or work colleagues, you will notice everyone has a different path to follow. They have their own goals, life, and aspirations. When it is time to follow your dreams, try not to listen to what they have to say. Their intentions may be good, but they don't know you like you know yourself. Most people will ask you to stick to the safe options. Safe options entail sticking to a secure job and education. They will ask you to get an education, get a good job, get married, have kids, and then retire. Let's say you want to leave your 9 to 5 job and open a restaurant. You will find many people give you advice and tell you how bad an idea it is. They will tell you not to leave the job. But you should go ahead and ignore what they say. Stay committed and true to your dream. Instead of sharing what you want to achieve, it is better to keep things to yourself and do what works for you. Remember, not everything you do will resonate with others. Most people are content being part of the rat race. They are used to society's standards and set on their ways. Some people don't like thinking out of the box.

Ignore Your Fears

People aren't the only ones who can stop you from achieving your dreams. You have to ignore what your deep-rooted fears say. They may make you think you cant achieve what you want. You may get terrified to fulfill your dreams. The challenging part is facing your fears, not allowing them to get in the way of your success. This quote by Eleanor Roosevelt describes facing your fears perfectly "You gain strength, courage, and confidence by every experience in which you stop to look fear in the face. You can say to yourself, 'I have lived through this horror. I can take the next thing that comes along.' You must do the thing you think you cannot do."

You have to get out of your comfort zone and grow as a person. Achieving your dreams is your way of growing as a person. Let go of your fears and learn to face them. Ask others for help if required. Support is important for us to thrive. Don't shy away from fears and hide in your comfort zone. Welcome them and thank them for making you stronger.

Ignore What Elders Have to Say

There is a big gap between you and your elders. What your elders think worked for them in the past may not work for you. They may have more experience, but it may not be in the same situation, and that's why you can't follow what your elders say blindly. If they want to offer you advice, listen to them, politely tell them you will consider it, and then do what you think is right. If you tell them about your dreams, they will always, without a doubt to be practical. That it is better to stick to what you know and ignore your dreams because they are for children. They may tell you about hypothetical roadblocks that you could face. They will discourage you and tell you that you will not be successful. All of these things are not true. No matter their seniority, most people won't understand your journey. Forget about what they have to say. If you don't follow your dreams, you will regret it. Only and only listen to your heart.

What Comfort Looks Like

Nobody has ever been successful while staying in their comfort zone. A lump of coal doesn't turn into a diamond without going through extreme temperatures. Similarly, you must be ready to step out of your comfort zone. Staying in one is a recipe for a dream killer because it can be so tempting. If you have a college degree, a decent job, and you're paying your bills, leaving all of it behind to pursue your dream may seem like a bad idea. But think about it; you may regret not being able to pursue it while you could. On your death bed, the comfort will have felt like you didn't do anything in life for yourself. You didn't push yourself, you didn't allow difficulties and problems to help you grow as a person, and, most importantly, you ignored your dreams and aspirations.

Conclusion

Dreams are born with you, and they are something different for everyone. They define your purpose in life, and no human being is complete without them. Many will discourage you from pursuing your dreams, but they couldn't be more wrong. Yes, you should accept all the support you can get, but ultimately, your heart's desires should take precedence over everybody else. Your dreams are a gateway to deeply understanding and knowing your true self. If you don't want to be one of those people who have deep regrets for not achieving what they wanted to in life, launch yourself into the path of your dreams and then watch yourself grow and flourish. Happy dreaming!

Disclaimer

This e-book has been written for information purposes only. Every effort has been made to make this eBook as complete and accurate as possible. However, there may be mistakes in typography or content.

The purpose of this eBook is to encourage people to invest in their lives and do things during their life that they can rejoice going back to their old age. The author and the publisher do not warrant that the information contained in this e-book is fully complete and shall not be responsible for any errors or omissions. The author and publisher shall have neither liability nor responsibility to any person or entity with respect to any loss or damage caused or alleged to be caused directly or indirectly by this e-book.

www.ingramcontent.com/pod-product-compliance
Ingram Content Group UK Ltd.
Pitfield, Milton Keynes, MK11 3LW, UK
UKHW041643190726
13854UKWH00006B/2663

9 789198 671704